SOLSTYCE NASSON

The Three Day Parasite Test

By Day Three You Will Know If You're A Host

*To my daughters Victoria and Shekinah, thank you for bringing me joy,
loving me tenaciously, and being so beautiful.
Love Always and Forever,
Mom*

Contents

1

Introduction

The Three-Day Parasite Test is part of a cleanse I first completed in 2018. By the third day, I knew I had them and so will you, if you have them. If you get a positive result, you can follow the protocol for an additional amount of time that is outlined later in the book or you can consult your doctor for medical advice. If you are among the fortunate people in the world that do not have parasites, then at least for Three-Days during the test you have tried something new and eaten super clean for Three-Days. :-) I did not consult a physician before I started the cleanse. I was just tired of feeling sick. I have suffered for over 45 years with eczema and dry skin. About 30 years ago I started retaining water that causes my feet to swell. I've had an allergy test for my skin, venous doppler for my circulation, stress test for my heart, I even went to a podiatrist to see if I had a broken bone in my foot that may be causing the swelling. My doctor told me I was obese for my height of 5"6'and my stomach sitting on my lap was probably causing a blockage in my circulation. At that time I weighed 186. When I told my husband what the Dr.said, he replied, "You are not fat, just wide." I carried the majority of my weight around my torso. A waistline? None Existent.

At the tender age of 19 my fingers started breaking out. The dermatologist told me to avoid dairy, peanut products, caffeine, tomato products, strawberries, mustard, smoked meats, corn products, and wheat. I replied, "Then what am I supposed to eat?" His answer was "Not these things." He suggested a Dietician but told me I would have to pay out of pocket cause my insurance did not cover it. I did not go to the dietician and managed my eczema with topical prescriptions as I was told it was chronic and I would have it for the rest of my life. When I was around 29 years old, I got my first Kenalog shot that cleared my eczema almost immediately. The result only lasted a few months so I got another one. After the 2nd shot, my dermatologist told me "I have to warn you, this shot is bad for your liver. Do you still want it? " I told her "No" she said "Good " and I continued to manage my eczema topically.

Fast forward a couple of decades later to November 2017. My diet had improved, but I was straddling the fence. I would eat well all week then on Friday order pizza with bacon and pepperoni. I was trying to be a vegan that only ate alkaline foods, drink spring water, and walk and run on the treadmill. I would try to drink up to a gallon of water a day but I was still using white white sugar AND French Vanilla creamer in my free coffee that I only drank at work. I would eat alkaline foods and food least detrimental to my system but then smash a bag of potato chips. In a nutshell, I was all over the place. My feet were still swelling, I was managing my eczema with creams but I felt horrible. Oh did I mention I was working out but still out of shape?

To battle my unshapeliness I got a waist sweat belt. My friend warned me that I was going to break out on my torso if I kept wearing it and I did eventually break out. I now know that my stomach and liver were so full of toxins that the sweat band was just pulling out toxins through my skin that were trapped in my digestive tract. When I went to the dermatologist, the PA looked at my torso and the expression on her face was like " you are Fawked up!" She gave me a prescription for the breakout on my torso and a list of over the counter products to use to assist my system. On that list was Psyllium Husk. In May of 2018, my oldest daughter suggested I do a parasite cleanse. I was working out, eating 80 percent clean, taking herbs, and drinking water but I still did not feel good nor was I looking my best. I tried and completed the cleanse. This book is a guide for you to test yourself for parasites and if you have them, show you how to kill them.

You purchased this book because you are serious about taking care of yourself. I created this book because I want to help you. During my annual physical in 2018 the Physician Assistant's response to my health inquiry was disappointing. I asked her, "could my chronic eczema and lymphedema be caused by parasites." The PA responded laughingly, "You don't live in a third world country." I responded " well I completed a cleanse a few months ago and I saw worms in my poop." She said " Really?" then offered to send me for lab work. I declined as I knew the natural products I used produced results. She referred me to a Cardiologist to determine the cause of my Lyphedema. The Lymphedema was more pronounced on my left lower extremity. Over the years, I've had a venous doppler, cat scan, and abdominal scan to confirm the cause of my lymphedema. But, a definitive cause was never found.

At my first visit with my cardiologist I asked him if I could have parasites. He said "probably not." I didn't mention my cleanse results and was told to schedule an Abdominal Scan. During my follow-up visit after my scan, I asked to see my scan results and the cardiologist asked me if I knew how to read a disk, did not show me my abdominal scan images, and told me to schedule another appointment. The test results were negative for heart disease so his diagnosis was "You must have an infection". When I asked "Where?" the cardiologist said " I don't know."

I scheduled another appointment. When I returned in two weeks, the PA rushed into the room like she was running from someone. Since no surgery was required, I was thrown into the hands of the Physician Assistant. After we discussed the history of my problems she blurted out "Oh well, you have Lymphedema, but there is no test for it." I was given a referral to the lymphedema clinic and advised to schedule an appointment for a lymphedema pump. I have yet to return to that cardiologist and I did not get the pump. My concern was getting to the source of my infection. My research told me that it was probably in my gut.

There are many cleanses on the market. I found a simple cleanse that after the first dose I felt movement in my digestive track and by the third day I felt wiggles in my anus then saw the parasites and eggs in my poop! All of the ingredients are plant based and were purchased from my local Health Food Store. To date, the supplements I use are not approved by the FDA to treat or cure diseases in America.

However, you will have either a positive or negative result. What you choose to do after day three is up to you.

I'm excited for you.
    Solstyce Nasson

2

What's Eating you?

Per the Center for Disease Control website a parasite is an organism that lives on or in a host organism and gets its food from or at the expense of its host. There are three main classes of parasites that can cause disease in humans: protozoa, helminths, and ectoparasites. Protozoa (Unicellular), Helminths (Multi-cellular), and Arthropods-Ticks and Insects. An infection from parasites can impact the human host emotionally, financially, socially and physically. A protocol to address severe cases is chemotherapy! However, we are addressing the issue with herbs, supplements, water and food for the test. The purpose of this book is to allow you to test and address the parasites with plant based herbs and supplements. The Three-Day Parasite Test will determine if you are infected with Helminths. "Helminth is a general term for a parasitic worm. The helminths include the Platyhelminthes or flatworms (flukes and tapeworms) and the Nematodes or roundworms. (World Health Organization 2014)

What is a Helminth and How Can You Get Infected?

Helminthiasis, also known as worm infection, is any macro parasitic disease of humans and other animals in which a part of the body is infected with parasitic worms, known as helminths. There are numerous species of these parasites, which are broadly classified into tapeworms, flukes, and roundworms.

Tapeworms come from eating undercooked beef, pork, and fish that is raw or not cooked to the proper temperature. That piece of fat on the end of your bacon that was not cooked to a crisp could be a source of tapeworm infection. The rare steak that is oh so juicy and tender could be your gateway to hosting a tapeworm. Flukes are transmitted to humans by eating raw or undercooked fish, crabs, or crayfish from areas where the parasite is found. The lifespan of flukes in the body can be a quarter of a century.

Roundworms include pinworms, whipworms, and hookworms. These parasites look like worms because they are and can be seen with the naked eye. Pinworms are spread by fecal oral transmission, that is by the transfer of infective pinworm eggs from the anus to someone's mouth, either directly by hand or indirectly through contaminated clothing, bedding, food, or other articles.

(Laura Bile 2018) states that 5% of the Amercan population is infected with Helminths. In 2018 5% of the population was 16.3 million Americans.

Millions of American children have been exposed to a parasite that could interfere with their breathing, liver function, eyesight and even intelligence. Yet few scientists have studied the infection in the United States, and most doctors are unaware of it. The parasites, roundworms of the genus Toxocara, live in the intestines of cats and dogs, especially strays. Microscopic eggs from Toxocara are shed in the animals' feces, contaminating yards, playgrounds and sandboxes. (Bile 2018)

(Daya) of Victoria Health estimates the number to be as high as 80 percent of the population is infected but that is in the UK. I argue that the infection rate could be as high as 90% globally with the remaining 10% of uninfected people addressing them properly with diet and herbal supplements.

You can get Helminths during an activity that I am notorious for and you may occasionally engage in: walking on your bare feet. Soil transmitted helminth infection can be transmitted from feral cats, dogs, and humans via their feces. Walking barefoot in contaminated soil is an invitation for the Helminth to attach itself to your feet, enter your body via a microscopic tear in your skin and start its journey into wreaking havoc. Although some people experience no symptoms, vomiting, abdominal pain, diarrhea, loss of appetite, visible worms in the stools, and weight loss are some of the symptoms present when helminths are present in the body. Helminths can also be passed by anyone that has the eggs on their hands and touch any surface like door knobs, phones, computer keyboards, gas station handles, etc. Additionally, you can get infected with parasites from any type of bug that feeds on blood. Lice, ticks, biting flies, fleas, and any other bug that bites the host and feeds off blood. People arriving from other countries and traveling throughout the world are sources of global transmission.

Some types of parasites are endemic to certain areas. Although mostly associated with tropical and subtropical locations they also can be found in Antarctica. Most common in Antarctica are lice, fleas, and mites. The species of penguins that nest in caves get fleas. Some types of parasites are endemic for certain locations. In the body, a parasite may involve a specific organ or travel through several organs. Cyst can be caused by parasites with rupturing causing severe infection.

Cysticercosis is a cyst caused after an individual swallows eggs of a tapeworm. The parasite then moves throughout the body and lodges in the muscle, brain and other tissues. In the brain, this infection can cause seizures. (World Health Organization 2022)

4

Where Do The Helminths Live?

Helminths live in the intestines and their eggs are passed in the feces of infected persons. They hatch and develop inside the small intestine and move to the large intestine as adults. Helminths can travel and live in your gut, blood, lymph, and tissues. Disease can be caused by the worm living in the gut, blood, lymphatic fluid, and tissues. As I suffer from Lymphedema,I think it is important to note that Lymphatic Filariasis is a parasitic disease that is more commonly known as Elephantiasis. The adult worms live exclusively in the Lymphatic system. Stage Stage 4 Lymphedema is elephantiasis which is also called Lymphatic Filariasis. Although typically noted in tropical and subtropical climates and thought to be endemic to these regions, global travel of the host could cause transmission in the America's. I am blessed that my lymphedema has not progressed to stage 4. In Endemic areas, chemotherapy is used to treat the parasitic infection in the blood.

Helminths have been seen beneath the skin of some individuals and proof that the worms travel throughout your body. During my first cleanse, by day three I felt the parasites moving in my brain. It can be argued that what you think is your bowels moving, it could actually be the parasites. Your irritable bowel syndrome could very well be parasitic infection. These arguments are strictly my own but I still argue it no less.

5

What Do Parasites Eat?

Parasites eat glucose or sugar. High carb foods like white sugar, white bread, pasta, rice and high sugar fruits are favorites of parasites. High sugar foods create an acidic environment in the body and help the parasites thrive. That sugar craving you have may not be you but the parasite craving the glucose. Parasites also eat the foods you eat and they may even eat you. External parasites, fleas, lice,ticks, and mites feed off your blood and deposit their larvae into your bloodstream. The parasites then deposit their larvae into your tissues, muscles, organs, and brain where they can cause a host of symptoms that could be confused with other diseases if not diagnosed properly. At that point you are literally the hostess with the mostest. :-(

6

Symptoms Of Parasitic Infection

Some diseases can have the same symptoms but could be from different causes or are they? For example unless specifically tested for parasites persistent gas could be thought to be caused by overeating. Swollen lymph nodes can be caused by a virus or bacteria. However, a parasitic infection from cat feces can cause swollen lymph nodes as well. One of the CDC TOP Five Parasites is Toxoplasma.

Toxoplasma is often called the "cat poop parasite," since it's frequently caused by close contact with a friendly feline. In the U.S., more than 60 million people are chronically infected with toxoplasma gondii. The parasite is also found in undercooked meat and even some unwashed fruits and vegetables. Health experts say toxoplasma can put pregnant women at risk for birth defects. Symptoms of this parasitic infection include swollen lymph nodes, muscle aches and eye complications. If left untreated these problems can become chronic. (Firger 2014)

Additional symptoms of parasitic infection are constant cough, anal itch, dizziness, insomnia, chronic fatigue, teeth grinding, iron deficiency, skin problems, rashes, eczema, acne, body odor, jaundice, brain fog.

Parasitic infections also share these symptoms:

- Nausea or vomiting
- Stomach cramps and pain.
- Dehydration.
- Weight loss.
- Digestive problems including unexplained constipation, diarrhea or persistent gas.
- Skin issues such as rashes, eczema, hives, and itching.
- Continuous muscle and joint pain.

7

Everyone Has Them, What's The Big Deal?

The thought of being the host to worms does not sit well with me. Parasites can travel throughout your body and could be the underlying cause of many diseases. If the thought of a piece of fruit having a worm is repulsive to you, then having worms in your body should be repulsive as well. That street taco you enjoyed in Mexico, that swim in Jamaica, the lush sands of Fiji, could all be the sources of infection. But you can also get them from that co-worker that loves cats and lets her cat walk on the kitchen counter but she makes a delicious cheese ball for every potluck.

You never know where you could pick up something. During my first cleanse I felt something moving around in my head, stomach, gut, and then saw them in my poop. To see the eggs was ultra distressing. To know I had these organisms and their eggs in my body was terrifying.. I'm not sure where I got them or how long I had them but I was glad that I was getting rid of them.

8

The Brain-Gut Connection

The enteric nervous system (ENS) is two thin layers of more than 100 million nerve cells lining your gastrointestinal tract from esophagus to rectum. A parasite that can affect the brain is the Pork tapeworm: Taenia solium. This parasite can cross the blood-brain barriers and travel to the central nervous system. The organism then develops into fluid-filled cysts and causes neurocysticercosis that results in seizures. Neurocysticercosis is one of five formidable parasitic infections. That little piece of chewy fat on the end of your bacon that did not fry to a crisp could very well be harboring an unwanted visitor.

9

Consult Your Doctor Before You Begin

As I am not a medical professional, I suggest you contact your physician prior to starting The Three-Day Parasite Test. The ingredients could interfere with certain medications. If you are pregnant, nursing, or trying to become pregnant, do not take this test or use these ingredients.

Beverages Allowed During The Three-Day Parasite Test

Water is essential to push the worms and eggs out of your body. Water will also help keep you hydrated and assist with proper bowel movements. I prefer to drink Spring water as well as Okra water. If you can splurge, drinking Alkaline water with a pH level of at least 8 or pH of 9 is optimal as it helps create an alkalinity in the body. Parasites thrive in acidic environments. Adding the juice of a fresh key lime if you can find them works well in boosting the alkalinity of bottled water. Key lime juice although acidic turns alkaline when consumed. If you can't find fresh key limes, I like to use about a teaspoon of Organic Pure Key Lime Juice to 16 ounces of water.

Fennel water made with Fennel seeds is a refreshing alternative to tea. When I lived in Phoenix Arizona, I would put a teaspoon of Fennel seeds in a 16 ounce mason jar, fill it with spring water and let it sit in the sun for a few hours. Natural coconut water is good but be careful not to consume too much as it is high in potassium and too much potassium can cause diarrhea. The best source of coconut water would come from a fresh coconut. Alternatively, you can make your own coconut water in a nut milk machine. I have an Almond Cow that I use to make coconut water. I like to use the cream that rises to the top from the coconut water made in my Almond Cow and add the cream to the fresh soup for dinner during the The Three-Day Parasite Test. These are the beverages that I chose to drink during the test just to keep things simple.

11

Beverages Not Allowed During The Three-Day Parasite Test

Alcoholic Beverages, Sodas (Reg or Diet), Coffee, Caffeinated Tea, Milk, Processed Beverages, flavored waters, energy drinks, any drink with sugar.

Foods Not Allowed During The Three-Day Parasite Test

For optimal results, do not consume any of the follow food.

- Sugar
- Agave
- Bread
- Pasta
- Meat
- Dairy Products
- White Rice
- Butter
- High sugar fruits like watermelon, grapes, mangos, dates, figs, prunes, any dried fruit
- Processed foods
- Potatoes

If the food did not come from the ground or a tree and has more than one ingredient do not eat it during The Three-Day Parasite Test. you can not eat chips, processed snacks, or nut butters with sugar.

13

Preparing For The Three-Day Parasite Test

I suggest you do a meal prep and prepare Three-Days worth of food to make sticking to the regimen easier. You may want to have your significant other and your family members join you due to the commonality of infection. Although I do not suggest you have children complete the test, in smaller quantities the cleanse ingredients may address any unknown pathogens in children. Parental discretion is advised.

The Shopping List below is what I used to complete the Three-Day Parasite Test.

14

Shopping List

Y ou will need 3 Meal Prep Containers for each salad and 3 Large containers to store the soups.

Ingredients: Parasite Test

- 3 Gallons of Spring Water*
- Liquid Bentonite Clay
- Food Grade Diatomaceous Earth
- Organic Lime Juice
- Black Walnut and Wormwood Oil (to kill the parasites)
- Clove Oil (to kill the eggs) or
- Parasite Cleanse Essential Oils (Oil Blend
- Shot glass (glass or disposable) or any small glass

*You will use one gallon of water per day for the parasite elixir, the cleansing cocktail, drinking to stay hydrated and help remove the toxins, breakfast smoothie, and making the fresh soup. For most people, drinking a gallon of water per day is okay. But if you have a condition that prohibits drinking a lot of water, talk to your doctor about water intake . The gallon of water consumption is spaced throughout the day.

Ingredients: Breakfast Smoothie

- 1 bag of frozen Berry Blend (For Breakfast Smoothie)
- Organic Lime Juice or 10 Key Lime or 3 Fresh Limes
- 3 Fresh Pears
- Tamarind (paste)

Optional Supplements:

- Sea Moss Gel or Sea Moss Pills (has 92 Minerals)
- Bladderwrack Capsules
- Burdock Root Capsules

For Snacks: 6 servings of low glycemic fruit like a pear, cherries, or grapefruit

- Walnuts or
- Raw Pepitas

* * *

Ingredients:Lunch Salad *Ingredients will be used for the Salad and/or the Soups

- Two to three heads of Romaine Lettuce
- Raw Pepitas about 1 cup
- Sliced Red Onion to your taste
- 3 Fresh Lemons
- Large White Onion (for soups)*
- Roma Tomatoes
- 2 Red Peppers*
- 2 Green Peppers*
- 2 Yellow Peppers*
- 2 Cucumbers
- Giardiniera (Optional 1 of 2 processed foods allowed)
- Fresh Lemon Juice for Dressing
- Private Selection Ranchera Salsa for dressing (If you just can't do Lemon Juice 2 of 2 processed food allowed)
- Oil of Oregano Supplement (Kills Bacteria)

* * *

Ingredients: Dinner Fresh Soup

- 1 small package of White Button Mushrooms
- 1 small package of Bella Mushrooms
- 2 cups of Butternut squash (1 Medium
- 3 cups chopped onion
- 3 cups chopped
- 3 cups of chopped peppers (blended)
- Fresh Squash) Frozen if you must
- 1 bulb of Fresh Roasted Garlic

- Grapeseed Oil
- 1 Bag of Dry Garbanzo Beans*
- I bunch of Celery with Leaves(if available)
- Baking Soda* (used to soak the lettuce)
- Vinegar (used to soak the lettuce)
- I bag of /dried Unsweetened Coconut Milk
- 16 Ounces of Seed Milk (if allergic to nuts)

Note each soup recipe will use at least 2 cups of nut or seed milk for a total of six cups for all recipes. Divide accordingly. Substitute as needed.

Herbs of your choice:

Fresh Thyme, Sage, Marjoram, Basil, or a bottle of Dried Italian Seasoning, Chili Powder, Bay Leave, Smoked Paprika, Paprika, Herbs de Provence, garlic and onion powder, or whatever herbs and seasoning you prefer to use to flavor your foods. These are just basic herbs, there are many more. If you choose to use packaged herbs, be certain to read the ingredients to make sure the herbs do not have additives like yeast and natural flavors as I am not sure what natural flavors include. It's best to check your pantry to see what herbs you have on hand before shopping.

* * *

15

Prepping the Garbanzo Beans:

This Step should be performed the night before Meal Prep as the garbanzo beans need to be sorted and soaked before cooking. You will need to sort the garbanzo beans to make sure there are no rocks or hard beans in the bag. If this is your first time sorting dried beans, I suggest you pour the beans onto a rimmed cookie sheet and go through the beans and pick out any rocks and dried up beans. Then place the sorted beans in a large bowl and cover with water, swirl the beans around to clean any dust and debris, and pour off that water. Add 6 to 8 cups of water to cover the beans. Add a pinch of baking soda to the beans to help soften the beans and de-gas them. Let the beans soak overnight or for at least eight hours. They will double in size. After soaking, pour off the soaking water. DO NOT BOIL THE BEANS IN THE SOAKING WATER.

* * *

Note: The cooked beans will be used for soup and some seasoned then air fried. Garbanzo beans are dry but they are the best beans as they are alkalizing to the body.

16

Clean and Prep Your Produce

Clean your kitchen sink. Add the three fresh pears, all veggies except for the lettuce, mushrooms, and onions - to the sink. Fill with cold water, add a few tablespoons of vinegar and sprinkle with baking soda, swirl around, cleaning the veggies with your hands or a soft cloth to remove debris, let sit for at least 15 minutes. Drain water. Refill the sink with water, add a tablespoon of lime juice, let sit for about 15 minutes. Drain. Produce is now ready for meal prep.

Remove the leaves from the romaine lettuce and rinse briefly to remove any dirt. Pat dry with a towel. Stack the leaves and slice crosswise. Thin slices are best. Add lettuce to a large bowl, fill the bowl with cold water to cover the lettuce. Add a tablespoon of vinegar, sprinkle some baking soda over the lettuce, swirl the lettuce around to mix and let sit for at least for 15 minutes.

Pour the water off the lettuce. Add more cold water for the 1st rinse. Let sit for 15 minutes

Pour the water off the lettuce. Fill a bowl of lettuce with cold water and pour a Tbsp lime juice into the water, swirl around,and let sit for at least 15 minutes. Drain/Pour off the water.

Tip: Get a salad spinner to remove excess water from cleaned lettuce to take your salad to restaurant quality.

If you don't have a salad spinner: Place about 4 large sheets of paper towels in a two gallon food storage bag and add the drained lettuce to the bag. You can gently move the bag to help drain the water to the towel. Carefully remove the paper towel from the lettuce and discard the paper towel. If the lettuce is still too wet, add four more paper towels and gently move the bag to help drain the water. The lettuce is now prepped for salad.

Mix ¼ cup each of the yellow, red, green peppers, and ½ cup sliced red onion to a bowl and store. Slice the peppers and remove the white pith, chop the peppers, set aside. Slice the celery length wise about three times, then chop . If you are lucky enough to get celery with leaves on top, get it. The leaves add an extra level of flavor. Chop the leaves into bite size pieces as you chop the celery. Set aside. Slice the white onion as thin as possible, set aside. Chop the mushrooms, set aside. Slice the red onion as thin as possible. Set aside. If you purchased the fresh butternut squash: Use a potato peeler to peel the skin off the squash. Cut about an inch off the top and the bottom. Cut squash squash in half, remove the seeds, cut in half. Cut the halves in half and cut into uniform cubs for roasting.

Tip: Get a Mandolin to slice the cucumbers and onions to slice as thinly as possible for the salad and soups.

Prepare Your Food

Garbanzo Beans- In an 8 quart pot pour the prepared garbanzo beans. Add 8 cups of water into the pot or a slow cooker (best option) add 1 Tbsp Italian Seasoning, 1 Tbsp of Onion powder, 1 Tbsp of Garlic powder, 1 Tbsp Sea Salt, bring to a boil. Reduce heat to low. Cover then simmer for an hour or until the water reduces to half way. Remove from heat and let cool. If using a slow cooker, simmer on low overnight or for at least 6 to 8 hours.

Fresh Pears: slice then chop the pears. Place in three separate sandwich bags and place in the freezer.

PREPARE THE VEGGIES FOR THE SOUP

HomeMade Stock: In two cups of water, simmer one bay leaf, two to three springs of thyme, chopped tops of celery with leaves, and only a pinch of salt, the ends of the white onion to make a broth to thin out the soup. Bring to a boil, reduce to low and Let simmer on low for about 30 minutes let cool.

Coconut Milk: In a high power blender take 1 cup unsweetened coconut shreds and 4 cups of water for creamy or 5 cups of water for regular and blend for about 5 minutes. Strain milk through a super fine strainer of a piece of folded cheese cloth. I have an Almond Cow nut and seed milk maker best investment ever,

Preheat the oven to 400.

Roasting the veggies for the soups is a good way to keep the prep simple and flavorful.

Cut the top off the three bulbs of garlic, to expose the tops of the garlic cloves, leaving the bottom stem intact, place in a piece of foil big enough to cover all three pieces, pour one teaspoon of grapeseed oil onto the top of the garlic of each bulb of garlic wrap in the foil, and place directly onto the oven rack and roast with veggies for the soups, until both are soft Check the garlic and squash every 20 minutes or so. Protecting your hands, gently squeeze the bulb to test for softness. It's done when it's soft and fragrant. If not soft to the squeeze roast up to an additional 15 to 20 minutes Roasting up to 45 minutesIt should be soft to the touch. Remove from the oven. Set aside as one bulb each will be used for the soups.

Mushroom soup: To a large bowl, add the 1 cup of the white onion, the chopped mushrooms, 1 cup of chopped celery, ⅓ cup each of the red, yellow, and green peppers, and one tbsp grape seed oil, a pinch of salt. Mix well. On two large cookie sheets spread the veggies so they are not touching. (if the pan is too crowded they will steam and not roast. Roast for 20 minutes, remove from the oven and mix then spread out evenly and continue to roast for about 10 more minutes, being careful not to burn. Let cool.

Butternut Squash Soup: to a bowl Add 1 cup white onions, 2 cups of cubed squash, ⅓ cup each of the red, yellow, green peppers, one tablespoon grapeseed oil and a pinch of salt. Mix well. On two large cookie sheets spread the veggies so they are not touching. (if the pan is too crowded they will steam and not roast. Roast for 20 minutes, remove from the oven and mix then spread out evenly and continue to roast for about 10 to 20 more minutes, being careful not to burn. Veggies should be soft, not burned. Let cool.

Mushroom Soup: ½ cup of stock to blender, add veggies, and one head of roasted garlic blend until smooth. Add milk to achieve desired consistency. You may or may not use the entire two cups, it's up to your taste, you want the soup to be creamy but still be able to taste the vegetables season to taste. Store in the fridge

Butternut Squash Soup: ½ cup of stock to blender, add veggies, and one head of the roasted garlic blend until smooth. Add milk to achieve desired consistency. You may or may not use the entire two cups, it's up to your taste, you want the soup to be creamy but still be able to taste the vegetables, season to taste. Store in the fridge

Garbanzo Bean Soup: Add a ½ cup of stock to the blender, with 2 cups garbanzo beans, 1 bulb of roasted garlic, 1 cup seed milk, seasonings of your choice, blend to desired consistency. Add seed milk to achieve desired consistency. It's up to your taste, you want the soup to be creamy but still be able to taste the vegetable, season to taste. Store in the fridge

Air Fried or or Oven Roasted Garbanzo Garbanzo Beans in a colander mix one teaspoon onion powder, one teaspoon garlic powder, 1 tsp liquid Aminos, and optional,1 drop of oil of oregano. Mix together then pour over the garbanzo beans. On the air fryer use the french fry setting and fry for up to 20 minutes, checking every 5 to minutes to prevent burning. Let cool and add to the Prepared Salad.

18

Breakfast Smoothie Recipe

To a high powered blender add:

    1 c Water (add more to your desired consistency the water should cover the fruit add more water if necessary)

1 c Frozen Berry Blend

1 bag of Frozen Pears

1 tsp Tamarind Paste

Blend until smooth and creamy and the tamarind is mixed well. Enjoy!

After the cleanse try adding a cup of frozen dark sweet cherries and thank me later.

Ingredients For The Test

The Parasite Cleanse Shot is a mixture of essential oils of Wormwood, Black Walnut, and Clove. The essential oil blends made of Wormwood, Black Walnut, and Clove kill the parasites and their eggs. There are many products on the market. I chose the essential oil as a personal preference.

1.5 oz. to 2 oz. of Spring Water mixed with 74 drops of the Parasite Cleanse Essential Oils. "Nature's Answer" Brand

Or

1.5 oz. to 2 oz. of water with 30 drops each of the Essential Oils of Black Walnut, Clove, and Wormwood.

Or if you have a Sprouts Market in your area get their brand of Parasite Cleanse Oil. Mix either brand with 2 ounces of Water.

Consult the label directions for dosage. I only used two ounces of water because the less water I used, the less I had to drink. Slam it back like a shot of Tequila because this shot is bitter.

After taking the first shot, you will feel the warmth of the oil moving through your digestive tract. You may feel some movement depending on your level of visitors. Wait one hour, two is best before drinking the

Cleansing Cocktails

20

Cleansing Cocktails

You will have two types of Cocktails three times per day made of natural detoxifiers and natural fiber. In the morning you will have the The OFGDE Cocktail, the BCP Cocktail midday and the evening cocktail will be the OFGDE cocktail again. The detoxificant cocktails will dry out and bind the parasites, bacteria, and fungi in the body. The natural fiber will help move the toxic sludge from your body. Chase each cocktail with 16 ounces of water.

OFGDE Cocktail- Organic Food Grade Diatomaceous Earth is the detoxificant to dry out and cut through parasites. The Fiber can be either Psyllium Husk Powder or Pills. If you have a wheat allergy try Slippery Elm Pills or Ground Flax Seeds.

OFGBC Cocktail- Organic Food Grade Bentonite Clay is the detoxificant to help pull heavy metals like lead and aluminum out of the system. Liquid Bentonite Clay and Psyllium Husk Cocktail. The Bentonite Clay will help pull the heavy metal toxins out of your system. Bentonite clay is negatively charged ions while Most forms of pollution, toxic chemicals, pet dander, pollen, mold, and other harmful chemicals in the air carry a positive electrical charge, making them positive ions.

(Holistic 2019)

Morning-OFGDE Cocktail

- 1 to 3 Teaspoon of Organic Food Grade Diatomaceous Earth
- 1 Tbsp of Psyllium Husk Powder or Slippery Elm Pills
- 8 to 16 ounces of water
- Tsp of Organic Lime Juice

Mix all ingredients together in a large cup and drink. The fiber will swell quickly so drink the cocktail quickly.

Midday-OFGBC Cocktail

Use Plastic spoons and glass or plastic to mix the Bentonite clay. Metal will deactivate the clays negative charge.

- 1 Tablespoon of Organic Food Grade Liquid Bentonite Clay.
- 1 Tablespoon of Natural Fiber
- 8 to 16 ounces of Water
- 1 Teaspoon Organic Lime Juice

Before use,shake the Organic Liquid Food Grade Bentonite Clay to mix. Mix all ingredients using a plastic spoon and cup. The fiber will swell quickly so drink the cocktail quickly.

Evening Cocktail:

- 1 to 3 Teaspoon of Organic Food Grade Diatomaceous Earth
- 1 Tbsp of Psyllium Husk Powder or Slippery Elm Pills
- 8 to 16 ounces of water
- Tsp of Organic Lime Juice

21

The Three-Day Test Protocol

Day One

- 5.am 1 Parasite Cleanse Shot
- 6.am 1 OFGDE Cocktail one hour after taking Parasite Cleanse Shot in 8 to 16 oz of water then drink another 16 Ozs of water, immediately after.
- 7 am Fruit Smoothie Tamrind Paste
- 8am 16 ounces of water
- 9am Snack Low Glycemic fruit, 2 to 3 tablespoons of Walnuts or Pepitas
- 10am 16 ounces of Water
- 11 am Lunch Salad with 1 Oil of Oregano Pill
- 12pm Parasite Cleanse Shot
- 1-2pm Bentonite Clay and Psyllium Husk Cocktail chased with 16 ounces of water
- 2-3pm Snack Low Glycemic Fruit about 7 Walnuts or 1/4 c of Pepitas
- 3-4pm 16 oz of water

- 5-6pm Soup with Fried Garbanzo beans as a garnish. 16 ozs of water
- 7 pm Parasite Cleanse Shot
- 8-pm Diatomaceous Earth Shot Two Teaspoons Mixed in 16 ounces water
- 9pm 8 ounces of Water and Sea Moss Capsules

Day Two

- 5.am 1 Parasite Cleanse Shot
- 6.am 1 OFGDE Cocktail one hour after taking Parasite Cleanse Shot in 8 to 16 oz of water then drink another 16 0zs of water, immediately after.
- 7 am Fruit Smoothie
- 8am 16 ounces of water
- 9am Snack Low Glycemic fruit, 2 to 3 tablespoons of Walnuts or 1/4 c of Pepitas
- 10am 16 ounces of Water
- 11 am Lunch Salad with 1 Oil of Oregano Pill
- 12pm Parasite Cleanse Shot
- 1-2pm Bentonite Clay and Psyllium Husk Cocktail chased with 16 ounces of water
- 2-3pm Snack Low Glycemic Fruit about 7 Walnuts or 1/4 c of Pepitas
- 3-4pm 16 oz of water
- 5-6pm Soup with Fried Garbanzo beans as a garnish. 16 ozs of water
- 7 pm Parasite Cleanse Shot
- 8-pm Diatomaceous Earth Shot Two Teaspoons Mixed in 16 ounces water
- 9pm 8 ounces of Water and Sea Moss Capsules

Day Three

- 5.am 1 Parasite Cleanse Shot
- 6.am 1 OFGDE Cocktail one hour after taking Parasite Cleanse Shot in 8 to 16 oz of water then drink another 16 Ozs of water, immediately after.
- 7 am Fruit Smoothie
- 8am 16 ounces of water
- 9am Snack Low Glycemic fruit, 2 to 3 tablespoons of Walnuts or 1/4 c of Pepitas
- 10am 16 ounces of Water
- 11 am Lunch Salad
- 12pm Parasite Cleanse Shot
- 1-2pm Bentonite Clay and Psyllium Husk Cocktail chased with 16 ounces of water
- 2-3pm Snack Low Glycemic Fruit about 7 Walnuts or 1/4 c of Pepitas
- 3-4pm 16 oz of water
- 5-6pm Soup with Fried Garbanzo beans as a garnish. 16 ozs of water
- 7 pm Parasite Cleanse Shot
- 8-pm Diatomaceous Earth Shot Two Teaspoons Mixed in 16 ounces water
- 9pm 8 ounces of Water and Sea Moss Capsules

22

Positive Test Result

Depending on your level of toxicity when you lay down to rest at night, if you have parasites you will feel them wiggling around your anus. They are dying so this is normal. You will feel movement wherever they are in your body. By day two you will see the worms in your poop and by day three you will see the eggs. At this point you have to decide if you want to continue or if you want to consult a medical professional.

If you continue to cleanse your body with the protocol after day 3: Continue the above Protocol for the next 11 days for a total of 14 days.

During Days 15-21 you will stop taking the parasite shot and cocktails but continue to follow the eating schedule, eat clean, with no sugar, flour, dairy or processed foods.

For the last week, day 22-28 you will resume the parasite shots and the cocktails, eat clean, following the daily schedule.

You can do a cleanse every six months.

23

Negative Test Result

Your body is a parasite pulverizer. Your immune system and lifestyle have been protected from these nasty invaders. Whatever you are doing, keep doing it! Please share your lifestyle tips with us on FaceBook.

24

Conclusion

If you have a positive test result, that is okay. You are not alone. Research indicates that almost everyone has parasites but could also have an illness that is linked to parasites but was improperly diagnosed. You have taken the first step into your journey into physical wellness. Consult with your doctor or medical professional and inform them of any herbs you're taking for contraindications of using herbal products with certain medications. Thank you for purchasing my book. If you have found this information helpful please leave a favorable review on Amazon. I value your support and feedback.

25

References

The Brain-Gut Connection. (2021, November 1). Johns Hopkins Medicine. Retrieved May 17, 2022, from https://www.hopkinsmedicine.org/health/wellness-and-prevention/the-brain-gut-connection

CBS News, & Firber, J. (2014, May 8). *CDC warns of common parasites plaguing millions in U.S.* CBS News. Retrieved May 17, 2022, from https://www.cbsnews.com/news/parasites-causing-infections-in-the-us-cdc-says/

Daya, S. (n.d.). *Most Of Us Have Intestinal Parasites.* Victoria Health. Retrieved May 17, 2022, from https://editorial.victoriahealth.com/most-of-us-have-intestinal-parasites

Parasites Liver Flukes. (n.d.). Www.Cdc.Gov. Retrieved May 16, 2022, from https://www.cdc.gov/parasites/liver_flukes/index.html#:~:text=Liver%20flukes%20infect%20the%20liver,the%20lifespan%20of%20the%20parasite

REFERENCES

World Health Organization. (2022, January 11). *Taeniasis/Cysticercosis.* Https://Www.Who.Int/. Retrieved May 16, 2022, from https://www.who.int/news-room/fact-sheets/detail/taeniasis-cysticercosis